HOW TO MAKE A GLUTEN-FREE DIET FOR BEGINNERS

LEARN ALL YOU NEED TO KNOW ABOUT CELIAC NUTRITION, DISCOVER GLUTEN-FREE FOODS

Jessy M. Brown

Table of Contents

INTRODUCTION

The fact that you have decided to read this book is proof that the gluten freedom movement is steadily increasing in popularity. People all over the world have decided that avoiding gluten was not just another diet option, but that it was absolutely crucial for the good of their health. This is not just another fad that will lose momentum before you even have time to investigate it and certainly is not another crazy shock diet. This change has been considered as one of the most practical ways for many people to lose weight, take charge of their health and start feeling like themselves again. But make no mistake, this diet is not for everyone.

Sticking to a gluten-free diet will take you down a path that can be seen as forged through adversity. The problem is that gluten is everywhere! Trying to eliminate an ingredient that is included in such a wide range of foods can cause some problems. The first challenge will be to find the willpower to stop eating enough of the food you've come to love. This is much easier said than done when the "healthier" substitute is not as tasty. The next challenge will be to learn how to get enough of the nutrients you need to stay healthy without compromising your decision to avoid gluten. And if that's not enough, most foods labeled "Gluten-Free" can be more expensive than their counterparts.

Whatever you decide, always remember that your body is your home. If you don't take the time to take care of it, where will you live? Taking the time to eat right, get enough rest, and exercise will always be best for you. Performing efficiently and at the highest level of your competence will only be possible if you take care of yourself. This may require a little more time and a little more effort, but it will certainly be worth it. Unfortunately, there is no "one size fits all" when it comes to our health and well-being. You have to get to work and assess your own needs. Never, never, never will you be able to spill from an empty cup. So believe me, take some time to find out what your body needs and you won't regret it.

By now, you should be wondering if all this fuss is worth it. And once again, I encourage you to think carefully about whether this diet is really right for you. This diet may not be exactly what you need. However, if it is, the benefits will far outweigh any challenges you face as a result of this decision. I hate to sound dramatic, but cutting Gluten from your diet can even save your life. So that you can be sure that this diet is right for you, please continue reading and learning more about Gluten and why avoiding it is so important. This may well end up being

one of the best decisions you've ever
made.

CHAPTER I
THE GLUTEN

Simply put, gluten is one of the proteins found in cereal grains such as wheat, rye, and barley. Gluten is produced by the combination of two different proteins. These proteins are Gliadin and Glutenin. The plant depends on its supply of Gluten because it serves as food for the plant during its development. When these grains are ground into flour, Gluten is responsible for the elasticity of the dough mixtures. It is this elasticity that gives our food a certain "chewing". People suffering from gluten intolerance are often encouraged to avoid oats as well. This is because oats can easily become contaminated with gluten-containing foods, as they are often processed in factories that produce food using wheat and other gluten-containing foods. Examples of gluten-free grains include millet, sorghum, brown rice, buckwheat, wild rice, quinoa and corn.

Wheat is often used to make the following foods:

- ✓ Bread
- ✓ Pasta
- ✓ Baking Products
- ✓ Sauces
- ✓ Cakes
- ✓ Soups
- ✓ Salad dressings
- ✓ Battered meat, poultry and fish
- ✓ Rye is used to make food like:
- ✓ Rye bread
- ✓ Cereals
- ✓ Beer
- ✓ Barley is often used to make:
- ✓ Beer
- ✓ Food coloring
- ✓ Yeast milk
- ✓ Malt milk
- ✓ Malt vinegar

✓ Soups

Many of the foods we eat may also contain some amount of Gluten as a result of being contaminated during the manufacturing process. These foods include:

✓ Dried Fruit
✓ Caramel
✓ Flavored coffee
✓ Food starch
✓ French fries
✓ Processed cheese and meat
✓ Vegetable and meat broth
✓ Bouillon cubes
✓ Dietary supplements such as multivitamins
✓ Ice cream

This list is not exhaustive. Time will not allow me to list all the foods that contain or do not contain Gluten and even if I had time, I would find it quite boring. The only effective way to determine if your food contains gluten is to read the label carefully. This will require a lot of your time for you to be accurate. This exhaustive process may not be suitable for everyone. The next chapter will help you determine if we are saying too much goodbye to anything.

CHAPTER II
WARNING: GLUTEN!

A recent survey highlighted that about one-third of all Americans are actively trying to remove gluten from their diet. This is a lot of people when we think of the fact that there are more than 325,000,000 people in the United States. But why are they making such a fuss? Let's take some time to examine some of the reasons many people have chosen to live gluten-free.

1. Celiac Disease

Studies have indicated that the number of individuals currently suffering from celiac disease is increasing. Although no official figures have been published, it is estimated that more than 1% of the world's population suffers from this disease. Celiac disease is especially common among the elderly. Worse still is the fact that many cases of people suffering from this disease have not been diagnosed. In fact, about 80% of people with celiac disease do not even know they have it.

But what exactly is celiac disease? As highlighted in the previous chapter, gluten is composed of two main proteins, gliadin and glutenin. Individuals with celiac disease react negatively to the Gliadin component. Celiac disease is classified as an autoimmune disease. This is because the immune system of these individuals will confuse Gluten with something dangerous like some kind of Bacteria. As a result, their bodies try to defend themselves against gluten and end up attacking themselves in the process. This attack can result in degeneration of the intestinal wall and can be fatal if left untreated.

Other symptoms of celiac disease

include:

- Nutritional deficiencies
- Anemia
- Chronic fatigue
- Vomiting
- Abdominal swelling
- Abdominal pain
- Diarrhea
- Digestive problems
- Decreased appetite
- Itchy rashes
- Irritability
- Depression
- Osteoporosis
- Damaged tooth enamel
- Joint pain
- Acid reflux

2. Sensitivity to gluten

Others, who do not suffer from celiac disease, have chosen to avoid gluten or eliminate it from their diet because they suffer from Gluten Sensitivity. These individuals may even have had a negative result when they did a blood test for celiacs, but they simply don't feel well when they eat gluten-containing foods. They may even suffer from symptoms that are quite similar to those of someone with celiac disease. Having Gluten Sensitivity means that the individual reacts negatively to Gluten even though their immune system is not attacking their bodies, as is the case with Celiac Disease. Symptoms of gluten sensitivity are usually not related to the gastrointestinal tract or cause any damage to the intestines. Rather, these individuals are more likely to experience fatigue, joint pain, abdominal pain, or even "brain fog. Fortunately, gluten sensitivity is not life-threatening.

3. Gluten Intolerance

Nor is gluten intolerance a threat to life. However, it will cause a great deal of discomfort. Individuals with this condition simply cannot process or digest foods containing gluten. This may be for a variety of reasons. That person's body may simply be unable to produce the enzyme needed to digest gluten-containing foods. Symptoms of gluten intolerance are often related to digestion and may include gas, bloating, diarrhea, or nausea. Just think of the result of consuming dairy products when you are lactose intolerant.

You should now be able to appreciate that living gluten-free is a very serious matter for some people and not a decision to be made lightly. You will appreciate the seriousness of the matter, especially if you also suffer from these symptoms. Chapter 3 of this book will highlight how to determine if you have any of the serious Gluten-related conditions that have been mentioned.

CHAPTER III
DISEASE DIAGNOSTICS

The biggest problem with the diagnosis of celiac disease, gluten sensitivity, or gluten intolerance is that the symptoms are very similar to those you would have if you suffered from other diseases. And because gluten is included in such a wide variety of foods, it's easy to confuse these ailments with your body simply reacting negatively to a particular type of food. That's why I would never encourage anyone to try to diagnose themselves. Celiac disease can be fatal if left untreated and if adequate measures are not taken to alleviate its effects.

Although Gluten Sensitivity and Intolerance are not life-threatening conditions, ignoring the symptoms can cause long-term damage to your body. Leave the tests to professionals. Think about how dangerous it would be if you diagnosed yourself as gluten intolerant when you actually have celiac disease. Even though you'll leave the final diagnosis to the professionals, it wouldn't hurt to learn more about the process.

Diagnosis of coeliac condition

A blood test is often used to confirm whether symptoms are the result of celiac disease. Remember that Celiac Disease results when your body confuses the Gluten protein known as Gliadin with a dangerous substance and attacks it. Your immune system is designed to produce a protein known as an antibody to fight any organism your body suspects is dangerous. This is also the case when you suffer from Celiac Disease. Your body will produce specific antibodies to defend against gluten. Therefore, blood tests are done to see if your body is producing the specific antibodies to fight gluten. Doctors often test for high levels of the antibody known as Transglutaminase Immunoglobulin A (IgA) antituberculose.

Diagnosis of gluten sensitivity or gluten intolerance

One of the easiest ways for doctors to determine if you suffer from Gluten Sensitivity or Gluten Intolerance is to ask you to remove Gluten from your diet for a period of approximately 30 days. If your symptoms disappear or become less significant during the time you avoid gluten, and these symptoms reappear when you reintroduce gluten into your diet, then it is obvious that your body is reacting negatively to gluten. A blood test can also be used to determine if you have any of these conditions.

Medical System Deficiencies

Gluten wasn't a big problem ten years ago. Doctors are much more concerned with improving their technique for diagnosing cancer and sexually transmitted diseases. Much less time is spent investigating negative responses to gluten consumption. As a result, even well-meaning doctors simply confuse the symptoms of intolerance to celiac disease or gluten with something else. Tests for celiac disease will probably be one of the last things your doctor will recommend. In addition, there have been a remarkable number of cases of doctors not diagnosing their patients' symptoms. Chapter 4 of this book will explain how you can help your doctor accurately diagnose your symptoms.

CHAPTER IV
HELPING YOUR DOCTOR

As highlighted in the previous chapter, your doctor is not perfect. I am not encouraging you to discredit any medical professional who has extensive training and years of experience. However, I encourage you to give them a hand. Approximately 10% to 15% of all diagnoses are incorrect. And despite the efforts of our doctors, this is also true in cases involving a negative reaction to gluten. Fortunately, there is much you can do to help your doctor make the best diagnosis.

Here are my suggestions:

Keep a food diary By now, it should be obvious that your symptoms are related to your diet. This is almost always the case when your symptoms are related to your gastrointestinal system. Keeping a food diary requires you to keep track of the foods you eat and how often you eat them. In an effort to be as accurate as possible, I also encourage you to keep track of how much you eat these foods. This type of information will give your doctor a clear idea of the type of food that may or may not be causing your symptoms. I encourage you to do this for about two weeks before your appointment. This will save you a lot of time because most doctors recommend that you keep an accurate food diary before you are diagnosed.

Your doctor may be empathetic, but he certainly can't literally feel your pain. They won't be able to make an accurate diagnosis if they can't isolate your symptoms. That's why you need to help them understand what you're feeling. Documenting your symptoms will be an invaluable gift to your doctor because it will help you rule out a series of unrelated illnesses in a matter of minutes. Make a list of all your symptoms and how often they appear. It would also be good to include if these symptoms occur at a specific time, such as when you engage in some form of physical activity.

Be as specific as possible. For example, don't tell your doctor that your stomach hurts. Where does the lower abdomen hurt? Is it a sharp pain? How long does the pain last? When was the last time you felt this pain? Anticipate the type of questions your doctor will need to ask and document the answers to the questions as accurately as possible. Providing this type of information will save you and your doctor a lot of time. Sometimes it's when we mention a specific symptom or a series of symptoms that help the doctor put together the puzzle of your illness. And don't we sometimes forget to mention some of our symptoms to our doctors? This will ensure that you will say everything you need to say without having to spend the whole day with your doctor.

Tell your doctor about other medical conditions

If you have other illnesses, you may have symptoms that may lead your doctor to make an incorrect diagnosis. Giving him or her the clearest understanding of your current medical condition is the best way to help you make the best diagnosis. It will also help your doctor not to waste time exploring treatments for a condition for which you have already received medication. It's also a good idea to give your doctor a list of your current medications. This will ensure that your doctor does not prescribe something that will react negatively to your current medication. Therefore, your doctor may need to adjust your current medication to treat any new conditions you have identified. Your doctor may also need to recommend some adjustments to your diet if gluten is actually affecting you negatively. You will need to have a clear idea of how adjusting your diet will affect how your body reacts to your current medication and make the best recommendation.

Tell your doctor about your family's medical history

Your family's medical history serves as a map of your own medical status. You will most likely suffer from ailments that are common among your family members. This is especially true of your parents, who are the most influential in your health. Don't be afraid to ask them. Our relatives, especially boys, may seem strong to our eyes, but learning about their illnesses can save theirs.

Be on Time for Your Appointment

Although this has nothing to do with it, I think it has to be said that we are often not too considerate of our doctor's time. Showing up late for an appointment will put your doctor in a very uncomfortable position. You will have to force him to wait or infringe another patient's time. In any case, this is a very inconsiderate act and I denounce it strongly. We are all very busy people. But deliberately wasting the time of the people responsible for saving lives is quite reprehensible. If you have to be late due to an unavoidable catastrophe, I recommend that you call the doctor's office and report it as soon as possible. This will give you enough time to carefully rearrange your schedule to accommodate other patients who may be waiting. The doctor may even use this time to take a well needed and certainly deserved rest.

Be patient Waiting for a diagnosis may seem like an eternity. Some have even described it as the longest wait of their lives. The minutes, hours or even days that may pass can be agonizing, but please be patient. Disturbing your doctor to make a decision will get you nowhere. Some things, like the queue of blood samples waiting to be analyzed in the lab, are simply out of your doctor's control. Allow them the time and peace of mind necessary to come to the most accurate conclusion.

So far, we've explored what gluten is, how it negatively affects some individuals, and even how to identify if it's hurting you. Next, we'll focus on the benefits of following a gluten-free diet.

CHAPTER V
THE GREAT BENEFITS OF LIVING GLUTEN-FREE

It goes without saying that eating a gluten-free diet will be very beneficial for those of us who suffer from the gluten-related diseases mentioned in the previous chapters. For some, this can be as simple as avoiding bumps and stomach pain or as severe as saving their lives. Whatever the case, the benefits will speak for themselves. But eating gluten-free goes far beyond helping us avoid any symptoms we may have when we consume gluten. Let's look at these benefits from a different perspective.

First, cutting gluten from your diet will force you to pay close attention to the foods you've been eating. Once someone decides to avoid gluten at all costs, they will have to start reading the labels and asking the relevant questions. As mentioned in Chapter 1, it's easy to identify foods that obviously contain gluten, such as bread, but how will you know if your nuts have been sprinkled with an ingredient that contains wheat to enhance flavor? Do you think restaurant owners and supermarket attendants will take your side when they think you're about to buy or consume something that contains gluten? Do you think they want you to stop buying their products? Of course not! Your life itself is in danger, so you should take all the necessary precautions.

Once you start examining the labels of the foods we eat a little more diligently, you will begin to see how terrible some of the ingredients in our foods are. Some foods contain harmful preservatives, artificial flavors, and chemicals that you would prefer not to eat. You will be surprised to see that gluten is not the only enemy in your food. These harmful additives are often carcinogenic or can cause serious damage to our body over time. These surprising discoveries will push you to look for organic alternatives and that's another benefit of the gluten-free diet.

The best option for this type of diet is to avoid over-processed foods. Most bread and pasta, for example, is made with bleached wheat and other dangerous substances. Many of the gluten-free alternatives will be made from healthier whole grains that have been processed enough to make the food pleasant, but not too much to keep as many nutrients in the food as possible. Excessively processed foods are also known to contain unhealthy oils. Therefore, a gluten-free diet, when given careful thought, will also help you avoid the multitude of illnesses associated with eating too many carbohydrates and overprocessed oils.

Many of those who have decided to follow a gluten-free diet have found themselves eating many more fresh fruits and vegetables than they would have eaten had they not followed this special diet. A diet rich in a blend of natural foods is always one that comes highly recommended. Consuming more fruits and vegetables will help strengthen your immune system and give you an incredible amount of energy to face each day. Eating such a healthy diet will also help you maintain a healthy body weight if you also take the time to exercise regularly and get enough rest.

People who are new to a particular diet often complain that they face the most temptation and the most challenges when they decide to go out to eat. Often, the waiter is too busy or uninformed to explain to you if your food contains gluten. In addition, cross-contamination is a very strong possibility in these situations and can pose a serious risk, especially for those with celiac disease. These problems become even more problematic when eaten as a group. You don't want to feel like the stranger and you certainly don't want to upset the waiter who will serve your food. As a result of these challenges, many Gluten Free enthusiasts have made the decision to eat less away from home. Eating at home more often will give these individuals total control over what they eat. Now you have the option of making delicious meals that won't have annoying side effects. I'm not encouraging you to be antisocial, I'm just explaining what has worked for others in our shoes. Also, eating home-cooked food will be very beneficial.

Benefits of eating at home:

    ✓ Save money
    ✓ Allows you to control the size of your food portions

✓ Excellent family bonding opportunities as food is prepared and consumed.

✓ You can be assured that your food is prepared in a sterile environment.

There is also some innovative research currently underway that shows a correlation between autism and gluten-free food consumption. Studies have shown that eating gluten-free has relieved the symptoms of autism in some children. There are still many conflicting reviews of research findings of this nature. However, it is quite remarkable that many children's hospitals have reported an improvement in the behavior and social skills of children with autism who have been switched to a gluten-free diet.

I have no doubt that eating gluten-free is a great idea if you have a gluten-related illness. Hopefully, you will also be convinced that this is a good idea for you too. However, please pay close attention to the warning in the next chapter of this book because, as with any decision, there are also disadvantages in cutting gluten from your diet.

CHAPTER VI
DANGERS OF EATING GLUTEN-FREE

One of the biggest problems when embarking on a gluten-free diet trip is that many of those who embark on this trip simply don't understand what they are getting into. They simply dive headlong into this decision, thinking it's just another weight loss diet fad or another healthy diet option. Although the benefits of this diet are obvious, you need to carefully evaluate if it is right for you. Even if you suffer from a professionally diagnosed gluten-related illness, you should think carefully about your next moves.

Two of the dangers associated with not carefully planning your gluten-free regimen that often stand out are:

1. Loss of essential nutrients

2. Eating unhealthy gluten-free foods

People who have decided to join the gluten-free regimen for any reason without carefully considering their options often end up losing key nutrients. Despite all the ailments or medical aspirations you may have about your ideal body, good health should always be our primary goal. It is impossible to stay healthy without a balanced diet. It is said that a person has a balanced diet when it takes time to consume the recommended amount of essential nutrients that our body needs daily. Consuming too much or too little of any one nutrient will not give you any long-term advantage, even if you achieve the goal of losing some excess weight.

The risk of becoming deficient in certain nutrients becomes very real for those who follow a gluten-free diet because they have significantly reduced their options.

Gluten is included in such a wide variety of foods that removing it from your diet will require drastic changes. Many of those who strive to avoid gluten are very busy people and have many conflicting responsibilities. This fast-paced world demands a lot of our time and we often have to sacrifice sleep to do everything we have to do. Eating a balanced diet was already very difficult and now you have decided to further complicate your routine by deciding to live gluten-free.

The result of this combination of having too much to do and not too many choices will result in one of three things. The individual may end up eating many gluten-free fast foods. They may also end up simply eating the same things over and over again. They may also end up giving up altogether. If you embarked on this trip because you have celiac disease or another gluten-related illness, quitting smoking is not an option. You have to find a way to make this diet work for the sake of your health and sometimes even your own life.

Unfortunately, the other options I mentioned weren't such good ideas either. Eating the same things over and over again will mean that you are consuming the same nutrients all the time. This type of monotony will make it very difficult to follow this diet because you simply won't enjoy eating the same thing so often. Eating the same foods all the time may not sound so bad, but think about the nutrients that are missing from the foods you eat. Sometimes it's that one missing nutrient in our diet that makes the difference in your health. For example, many gluten-free bread substitutes often use alternatives to wheat that contain much less dietary fiber. Dietary supplements may help alleviate the effects of such dietary habits, but it is never the most recommended option. It will take a certain amount of planning on your part to get the right mix of nutrients.

Another big challenge that many people face when deciding to live gluten-free is that they get confused about the types of foods that are actually beneficial to their health. Because this movement is gaining momentum, furtive marketing executives have been labeling everything gluten-free. I've even seen "Gluten Free" labels on water bottles. You read that correctly - they're trying to sell gluten-free water! As funny as that may sound, this is a serious problem. Sending such a misleading message can only harm consumers.

To make matters worse, many of the foods sold gluten-free are actually very bad for your health. In order to make these foods tastier, producers often include a lot of fat or sugar. Many of these gluten-free foods are often overprocessed as well. That's why I can't stress enough how important it is that you read the labels of everything you eat. Check the caloric, fat and sugar content of each item. Don't make the mistake of assuming that these items are good for your health simply because they're labeled 'Gluten-Free. As highlighted in a previous chapter, you have to look out for your own interests. These sneaky providers often don't consider your best interests.

This information is in no way designed to scare you. But your health is a very serious matter. If you're not careful, your life could be at stake. You can never be too careful about what you put in your body. Take extreme caution with anything you intend to eat, no matter how nutritious it seems. Take the time to research anything new or that may seem questionable. If in doubt, follow the natural alternatives. You can never go wrong with fresh fruits, soil provisions and vegetables. But it can be very difficult to figure out how to enjoy eating natural foods. That's why the final chapter will give you some simple recipes to help you get started.

CHAPTER VII
HOW TO ENJOY EATING GLUTEN-FREE?

Eating a gluten-free diet doesn't have to be boring. As noted above, following any diet will become more cumbersome if you force yourself to eat the same things over and over again. This will not motivate you to continue with your diet. And the moment you see something that looks a bit like a challenge, you'll give up. Unfortunately, quitting smoking is not an option if you have celiac disease, gluten sensitivity, or gluten intolerance. Your health and your life are in danger and you need to move on.

Here are my suggestions for keeping you motivated to follow this

diet:

1. Mix it all up! This is the number one step to enjoying your gluten-free journey. Don't be afraid to try new things. If in doubt, read the label or research online. Once you're sure it's gluten-free, start eating! Include it in the meals you already enjoy. Mixing it will also require you to try new recipes. Your meals should be like a work of art. This doesn't mean they have to be elaborate, they just have to be eye-catching. Incorporate a variety of different colors, flavors and textures. Don't be alarmed if you fail a few times before you get it right. This is all part of the adventure.

2. Don't cut the carbohydrates! This may seem like a logical step to include in any diet. However, that's when you make the mistake of assuming that eating gluten-free is like any other diet. Always remember that your goal is simply to avoid gluten-containing foods. Carbohydrates are not the enemy. Once you've done your research to determine that the food is safe, dig and throw it away.

3. Beyond my suggestion that you `buy', I also strongly recommend that you treat yourself and eat yourself once in a while. This is another way to avoid making this diet feel boring or onerous. Gluten-free treats are very easy to find and just as enjoyable. Now that your options are a little more limited, you may also want to consider several fruits and nuts as a treat. Dried fruits and yogurt treats, for example, are simply divine and there are many more options to choose from. You might even include options like these like regular snacks between meals.

4. Don't starve! This new diet won't require you to eat fewer calories a day. Please don't starve to death. You may even find yourself eating a little more. Some gluten-free alternatives, especially those made from natural ingredients, often contain far fewer calories than we are used to. The result is that we will need to eat a little more of these foods to feel satisfied. Again, there's no shame in once the research has been done to determine that this food is safe.

5. Don't be shy! There's no need to be shy about eating gluten-free. Speak up and tell your friends, family and even the waiter who serves you that you have chosen this diet and explain the seriousness of your decision. Once they understand the gravity of the situation, they will also become very vigilant and help you monitor the foods you eat as well. They will cover your back and serve as an extra pair of eyes. Remember, two heads are better than one. And believe me, it's always better to tell the truth than to try to hide your illness or your decision. You'll seem pretty strange when you start avoiding the foods you once loved. Your friends might even worry a little and assume that you are one of those dangerous shock diets. Calmly explaining the logic behind your choice will gain your trust and support.

What you should learn from this chapter is that living gluten-free can be fun and exciting. Think of it as a new and challenging food journey. You will dare to leave your comfort zone and explore an unknown territory. Some have even described diet as a way to feel more in control of their lives and are thrilled to have developed such amazing self-discipline. Why should it be any different? Developing the discipline needed to remove gluten from your diet can give you the inner strength needed to take charge of your life in other ways as well. Whatever the case, enjoy the trip. The next chapter will help you learn a little more about the foods you can eat.

CHAPTER VIII
WHAT CAN YOU EAT?

Don't make the mistake of assuming that once you switch to a gluten-free diet your life is over. Even if you are a food lover, you can enjoy a wide variety of delicious and, of course, nutritious meals as well. All you have to do is change your perspective. Instead of looking around and imagining the obstacles, look at all the new possibilities. This is an opportunity for you to learn to be more selective and creative with your food. First, take a look at all the things you can eat with complete confidence that they do not contain gluten:

- ✓ Unprocessed Beans
- ✓ Unprocessed seeds (e.g., chia seeds, flax and pumpkin seeds)

- ✓ Vegetables
- ✓ Raw walnuts
- ✓ Eggs
- ✓ Most dairy products
- ✓ Meat
- ✓ Fish
- ✓ Poultry
- ✓ Fruit
- ✓ Gluten-free flours (can be potato, bean, rice, soy or corn).
- ✓ Dominican Corn
- ✓ Quinoa
- ✓ Tapioca
- ✓ Millet
- ✓ Potatoes
- ✓ Olive oil
- ✓ Coconut oil
- ✓ Ghee
- ✓ Sorghum
- ✓ Rice pudding
- ✓ Soy
- ✓ Teff
- ✓ Cider
- ✓ Wine
- ✓ Jerez

- ✓ Port
- ✓ Alternatives to bread products:
- ✓ Millet chia bread
- ✓ Brown Rice Bread
- ✓ Red rice bread from Bhutan
- ✓ Chapata bread Alternatives to pasta:
- ✓ Quinoa Pasta
- ✓ Corn spaghetti
- ✓ Spaghetti with Riso
- ✓ Penne rice flour

Although these foods are naturally gluten-free, you still need to be cautious. This is especially true if you have not prepared the meal yourself. You still need to pay attention to the amount of calories you eat and the amount of sugar and fat you are eating. Please remember that not everything that is labeled gluten-free is really good for you. Avoid any meat, fish or poultry that has been marinated, covered, breaded or battered. You can never be sure what they included in that mix. It would also be a good idea to avoid processed legumes and nuts or carefully read labels before eating them. You can never be sure what was used to enhance flavor.

Fortunately, eating out is still an option. Because of all the attention the gluten-free diet is receiving, several gluten-free restaurants have been popping up. Do a quick Google search to try to identify if there are any in or near your community. You might even consider starting a business on your own as well. Gluten-free dinners or even gluten-free support groups will attract people to your establishment.

Your gluten-free diet will affect every area of your life. Please try to remember that some medications also contain gluten. If you are visiting a new doctor, be sure to explain that you have removed gluten from your diet and the reasons for doing so. It's also obvious that you'll have to read over-the-counter medicine labels very carefully.

CHAPTER IX
SOME FOOD
PREPARATIONS

Start with a simple 7-day meal plan. There's no need to try to solve it all at once. You have time. Think about the foods you already enjoy, identify all possible sources of gluten and try to eliminate them. Start simple and then progress from there.

How about this:

Monday

✓ **Breakfast:** French fries and scrambled eggs
✓ **Lunch:** Creamy potato salad with cashew nuts

✓ **Dinner:** Eggplant steak with garlic and ginger and sweet potato pieces

Tuesday

✓ **Breakfast:** Banana and walnut Gluten-free pancakes with mixed berry topping and agave syrup
✓ **Lunch:** Gluten-free burger with bacon
✓ **Dinner:** Meatballs and butter bean stew

Wednesday

✓ **Breakfast:** Berry shake for breakfast with fruits of your choice
✓ **Lunch:** chopped BLT Salad
✓ **Dinner:** Gluten-free chicken cake

Thursday

✓ **Breakfast:** Breakfast hashish with sweet potatoes, ham and eggs
✓ **Lunch:** Gluten-free quinoa burger

✓ **Dinner:** Grilled salmon with cilantro rice

Friday

✓ **Breakfast:** Acai bowl with banana berry topping
✓ **Lunch:** Gluten-free fish tacos with avocado and Mexican cheese
✓ **Dinner:** Gluten-free chicken and dumplings

Saturday

✓ **Breakfast:** Potato frittata and broccoli
✓ **Lunch:** Chicken Chili with Cheese
✓ **Dinner:** Garlic chicken with rice noodles

Sunday

✓ **Breakfast:** Baked potatoes with tuna and caramelized onions
✓ **Lunch:** Turkey burger made with zucchini muffins
✓ **Dinner:** Shrimp Burrito Bowl

Everything I just listed in Gluten Free. These recipes include things we already do at home. All you need to do is take some time to research the gluten-free alternatives to the bread and pasta we're used to. Again, the key is to keep the fun and move on. Eating a gluten-free diet doesn't have to be complicated. The best part is that making a gluten-free meal doesn't always have to consume a lot of your valuable time. All you need to do is plan ahead and get some of the preparation done ahead of time. Vegetables can be chopped and refrigerated during the week. You can even set aside your day off to prepare the meal and simply reheat it as the week progresses. There's no need to interrupt your routine - find out what works for you and stick to it!

CONCLUSION

My intention was to give you the most realistic view of the gluten-free diet. Hopefully, you should be able to determine if the gluten-free diet is right for you or not. What I hope you've gotten out of this book is that if you don't have a diagnosed gluten-related illness, this may not be the best diet for you. If you are trying to lose weight, there are many other alternatives that include reducing your calorie intake and getting more exercise. But if you decide to continue on this journey, please remember to be cautious.

If you suffer from celiac disease, gluten intolerance or gluten sensitivity, I hope you found my suggestions helpful. While the benefits of this diet are obvious, I know you face many challenges. But there's no shame in asking for help. Involve your family and friends. The support of your loved ones will give you the energy you will need to move forward. You might even join a support group. While it's good to have loved ones encourage you, it would be even better to look for people who understand what you're going through. You could meet in person or even on social media and share recipes and experiences.

Whether or not you have celiac disease, you have to move on. Your health is a very serious matter and you should not take these diseases lightly. I don't want to scare you, but some of the symptoms associated with these diseases can be fatal. Remember that the first step to recovery is for a medical professional to examine your symptoms. It's always best to know how serious your condition is. There are some situations where simply adjusting your diet won't be enough. You may also need other medications. Take the recommendations in Chapter 4 very seriously because these suggestions could make a difference in whether or not your doctor makes the right diagnosis.

In conclusion, please never be embarrassed by your diagnosis. Please don't be fooled by all the rubbish that these dishonest people have labeled gluten-free. And finally, please enjoy this new journey no matter what challenges you face.

Remember that theory without practice won't do you any good, take whatever you learn into action.

I wish you the best in your results.

A big hug, your friend, Jessy!

By the way, I highly recommend you, if you want to learn a lot more about how to improve your health, my book on "BASIC ESSENTIAL FOODS FOR GOOD FOODS" is a book that I am sure will help you a lot on your way to "good nutrition".

Without further ado, you can find it on the Amazon search engine, by title or by searching for my name, such as: "Jessy M. Brown". Once again, I wish you success in your results!

www.ingramcontent.com/pod-product-compliance
Lightning Source LLC
Chambersburg PA
CBHW070441290526
45791CB00005B/2061